GIVE THANKS
RELEASING GOD'S ~~

November is the month of Thanksgiving and
the year is good for growing in giving thanks!
and makes you whole! Thanksgiving is high-l~
good! Thanksgiving is the way to God's heart ~
light and have fellowship with Him, the way to ~~~~~~~~~~~~~~~~ ~~ ... the
and making it whole, the way to defeat your ene~~~~~~~~~~~~ ...~ ~~ cleansing your soul
with a willing mind. Along with thanksgiving, yo~ ~... also have easy to do healthy eating and water
challenges that will improve your health, and set you up for a healthier life! Food is medicine to your
body and soul, and water brings many blessings to your health!

Each day you will read a thanksgiving devotional and answer questions that feed your soul on the
healing word of God. Coming to God's word is not about figuring things out, but meeting with Him and
letting Him teach and heal you. He wants to fellowship and have a personal relationship with you. He
wants to talk to you, lift you up, and help you. The Holy Spirit is your helper, teacher, counselor, and
comforter, so every time you come to the word of God, pray and ask Him to meet with you and speak to
you. Ask Him things that you don't understand and take time to listen to His voice. He'll amaze you as
He brings the Truth alive to you personally. As you draw near to God through His word, thanksgiving,
and praise, you will be filled with His Spirit's love and become new! You'll have short affirmations to
use through your day so you can abide in Him and experience Him.

Each week as you go through the healthy eating and water challenges, you will focus only on one thing
at a time, gaining momentum as you go through the three weeks. Start out the first week focusing only
on drinking at least eight 8oz. glasses of water while eating your normal diet. That week you will have
water tips to motivate you each day. The second week, you will continue your 8 glasses of water and
add a green smoothie. These are very simple to make with just greens and fresh fruit. You will have
living food tips to inspire you each day through that week. The third week you will continue your eight
glasses of water and smoothies and add a vegetable bean soup for lunch. That week you will have daily
thanksgiving quotes to encourage you each day to give thanks in everything.

These simple yet powerful tools to good health through drinking water, enjoying whole food, and giving
thanks will guide you to living a very healthy and happy life! Giving thanks to God fills you up with the
love and mercy that God has for you! This fills your heart with gratitude and changes your entire
perspective to good, which brings so much change for the good! Your soul will feed on God's goodness
and experience many wonderful and amazing blessings. Not only will you overflow with good things
through God's power for life and thanksgiving, but I guarantee that your relationships will come alive
and become miraculously good as you learn and practice thanksgiving daily! Giving thanks is a win win
in every area of your life!

You could take this 21 day thanksgiving whole health challenge and enjoy it with your spouse or
children, as a family, or even with a friend. You could set a time to meet each day, every other day, or
once a week, whether on the phone or in person. You could also do this with a group, and everyone who
is participating can share through email to encourage one another, or you can all get together once a
week. Your thoughts and words matter and help stir others on, and so do theirs to you, so doing this
with others will increase your motivation and blessings.

HUMILITY:

GIVE THANKS
RELEASING GOD'S POWER TO BE WHOLE

God came to bestow on you, to clothe you, with His beauty, His righteousness, His love, His truth, and His Spirit. His Spirit is a Spirit of humility and faith; humble and faith filled people are overflowing with thanksgiving. Coming to know Jesus and following Him means denying yourself and not doing things apart from Him; it requires complete dependence on Christ to do all things through you. Humility means believing the word of God over what you feel, see, hear, or experience, and receiving and experiencing God's abundance of grace. Grace is God's supply. He will meet your need. Trying to meet your own needs is prideful, and allows the devil to remain and resist God. Humbling yourself to believing the word is drawing near to God and having Him draw near to you. "Therefore submit to God. Resist the devil and he will flee from you. Draw near to God and He will draw near to you… Humble yourselves in the sight of the Lord, and He will lift you up." (James 4:7-8, 10)

Humble people are easy to get along with, excellent forgivers, teachable, helpful, thankful, loving, kind, and bring joy and peace wherever they go. Jesus was humble and gentle, and whatever you do in the name of Jesus is to be done with humility and gentleness. Humility is God's wisdom to make you beautiful, victorious, and to bring you favor, honor, and glory. "Wisdom will exalt you when you exalt her truth. She will lead you to honor and favor when you live your life by her insights. You will be adorned with beauty and grace and wisdom's glory will wrap itself around you, making you victorious in the race." (Prov. 4:8-10 TPT)

Humility is God's way to lift you up and pride is the devil's way to push you down. Choosing life is choosing to be humble. Humility will make you a winner, but pride a loser. Humility makes you a positive person who sees good in every situation and prays blessings for everyone. Ungodliness is caused by thanklessness. Unthankful people feel entitled and live comparing themselves to others and judging others. Thankful people feel blessed to have what they have and rejoice in God's salvation daily, and are givers wherever they go, considering others better than themselves. They are extremely thankful to God for the indescribable gift of Jesus that supplies for all their needs. Not being thankful to God makes your heart dark and your mind futile. It's a disease, and God has given you the remedy by putting His Spirit of love and truth in you to give thanks in everything and live through Him.

Thanklessness is very dangerous to your mind, soul, heart, body, and life! Being thankful, though, is the way of safety, protection, provision, and all the good and perfect gifts in life that God has for you. Being thankful and giving thanks in everything does not come naturally for anyone. That's the reason for this book. The purpose of this book is to help you to train yourself up in thanksgiving so that you can enjoy God, others, and all His rich blessings for your life. To be thankful is to simply focus your eyes on Jesus, coming to Him daily with a grateful heart expressing thanks for His blood that delivered you out of sin and bondage, and gave you life more abundantly. This is your new life in Christ, so come taste and see that the Lord is good and begin daily to rejoice in His work on the cross to redeem you!

When practicing God's love all day by giving Him thanks, you will live by faith and be blessed. You receive all things by grace, God's supply, through faith. You've practiced worry, anxiety, and fear and you've practiced it in your home, at work, at the grocery store, while driving, walking, watching TV, and maybe other places. You know how to practice these; therefore you can easily practice God's love, truth, and mercy just as successfully in all those ways and places instead, and can enjoy God's peace and power through giving thanks to Him. You have a choice every day to practice fear or love. Choosing to practice God's love or Satan's fear is something you do daily by the words you think, speak, and believe. Your tongue really does have the power of life and death and it is steering your whole life, so by giving thanks in everything, Jesus is guiding your life. You have all the power you need in Christ, so as you simply give thanks daily for God's creation, truth, people, things, even problems, all things, you will be made very healthy and free. God wants to fully satisfy you with His love and prosper you in all things and in health, and He does this as you put your focus on Him and give thanks in everything. He will lavish you with His great love, fill you with His power and strength, and fully satisfy you as you practice giving thanks in everything. Christ rules your heart and life as you give thanks always and living in Him gives you an abundant life!

Thoughts direct your ways and God's thoughts and ways of giving thanks in everything are high, perfect thoughts and ways that bring you rich blessings. Simply changing your thoughts and words to thanksgiving will always lead to good, and will automatically change your ways to good. You are able to change the way you eat and live by God's way of thanksgiving. You are replacing the old thoughts and ways for God's and wonderful changes will come automatically. His Word will provide and turn whatever is wrong in you to what is right. His Word is living and powerful, life and peace, and it will heal and deliver you.

Your new language as a new creation in Christ leads to God's good plan for you. His way of thanksgiving makes you see things differently, in a good way, and gives you a new life full of God's goodness!

I have prayed many blessings over you! I believe in the power of prayer and expect God to help you succeed in accomplishing these simple things and lead you to an abundant life! If you are in for more of a challenge, go through this book again, drinking ten glasses of water daily and filling 75% of the blender with greens, a handful of raw almonds, and a half cup of flax seed or Chia, the other 25% with fresh fruit. Fill your entire 64oz. blender and drink your smoothie all through your day. Then have your soup for dinner with quinoa or rice, along with a salad made with your favorite vegetables and home made avocado dressing. Avocado, tomato, and lemon (option: add fresh cilantro or other herb you like) in the blender makes a tasty, healthy dressing. I assure you that you will be a different person each time you reach the end of this book, and will experience wonderful changes in every area of your life!

THREE FOOD AND WATER CHALLENGES
For the first 7 days you will start drinking eight, 8oz. glasses of water daily. During the second 7 days you will start drinking a green smoothie daily. Use any greens, like kale, romaine, spinach, collard, or chard and add fresh fruit of your choice. Fill half the blender with greens and half with fruit. Super simple and very delicious! During the third 7 days you will start making a vegetable bean soup to have daily for lunch.

God made you to smile, be joyful, thankful, and live in Him. So smile, shine His glory, and give thanks to people everyday!
- Smile, shine God's glory, and give thanks to people for something at least 3x a day the first 7 days.
- Smile, shine God's glory, and give thanks to people for something at least 4x a day the second days.
- Smile, shine God's glory, and give thanks to people for something at least 5x a day the third 7 days.

21 DAYS OF THANKSGIVING CHALLENGES
Every time you drink water
Thank You, God, for using this water to bless my body and make it healthy.
Every time you have food
Thank You, God, for giving me new desires for healthy food and using this healthy food to bless me

with great health, body and soul.

Every day say out loud

"Thank You, God, for _____ (specific things for which you are thankful for your spouse, children, parents, or those closest to you)." "Thank You, God, for filling my heart with gratitude and love for You and others, and for helping me to express words of thankfulness in every situation!"

"I'm taking the way of life and peace. I am a thankful person. I give thanks in everything."

Every day thank God for things He has created

Romans 1:21 "Although they knew God (as the Creator), they did not honor Him as God or give thanks (for His wondrous creation), but became futile in their thoughts, and their foolish hearts were darkened.

Write down one thing a day that God created that you are thankful for and tell Him why you are thankful for it.

Remembering that God is your Creator and made all things is critical to living a healthy life. Giving Him thanks daily for His creation will keep you thankful for all He's made for you to enjoy.

Say out loud or silently, anytime and as many times as necessary, to receive peace in difficulty

I have the way of escape in every trying situation. I say, "Thank You, Lord, for using all this mess for so much good in my life. Use it all, God." (Rom.8:28)

Say the daily verses out loud

You will have daily Scripture verses to say, with questions to help you meditate on them.

Pray with thanks to God daily for His love, and release His power of love in your family

Thank You, God, for binding me, my spouse, and children to You and tightly together in Your love. Thank You for teaching us how to love each other in every situation, and show kindness and grace.

The Thanksgiving Key

You can either make a key out of card stock or use a real key. Write on it 'Thankful'. Put that key in front of you constantly throughout these 21 days. Put it on your table when you eat, on your table when you watch TV, or on your vanity when you get ready. Make it visible throughout the day and watch yourself overcome, find victory, and be blessed in every way! You may make more than one key and place them in specific, strategic places.

Day 1

Pray and ask the Lord to speak to you. Read these verses out loud then answer the questions.

Make sure that nobody pays back wrong for wrong, but always strive to do what is good for each other and for everyone else. Rejoice always, pray continually, give thanks in all circumstances; for this is God's will for you in Christ Jesus. Hold on to what is good... May God himself, the God of peace, sanctify you through and through. May your whole spirit, soul and body be kept blameless at the coming of our Lord Jesus. The one who calls you is faithful, and he (Christ) will do it. (1 Thess. 5:15-18, 21, 23-34) "Death and life are in the power of the tongue, and those who love it will eat its fruit." (Prov. 18:21) "Listen carefully to Me, and eat what is good, and let your soul delight itself in abundance. Incline your ear, and come to Me. Hear, and your soul shall live. (Isa. 55:2-3)

- **Why doesn't God want us to repay wrong for wrong? What is God's solution when someone does something wrong to us?**
- **What is God's will for your life?**
- **Why is that God's will?**

- How intentional are you in doing God's will?
- How important is your attitude and response when difficulty comes?
- What are the amazing blessings you will receive from God by doing His will in all circumstances as you give thanks?
- What are the many issues you will experience in your life as well as your spirit, soul, and body when you're not giving thanks according to God's will, but arguing or complaining?
- What is good that God wants you to cling to, and what is evil that He wants you to reject?
- How do you become whole (healthy) spirit, soul, and body?
- Where is the power you need for life, wholeness, and peace?
- What do the words you listen to and speak have to do with your life?
- What does sanctify mean?
- How do you see the goodness and love of God through these verses?

AS YOU GO

As you go through your day, focus your mind on all the amazing blessings you receive by doing God's will and giving thanks in everything. Smile, shine God's glory, and give thanks to people for something at least 3x a day.

AFFIRMATION

I will give thanks in all circumstances, for this is God's will for me in Christ Jesus to fill me with His peace and make me whole!

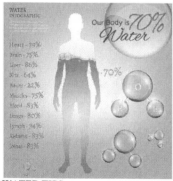

WATER TIPS

Whoever drinks of the water I will give them will never thirst. Indeed, the water I give them will become in them a spring of water welling up to eternal life. (John 4:14)

Maintain a healthy pH and electrolyte balance by staying hydrated! Water helps keep your body temperature normal. It also lubricates and cushions joints, protects your spinal cord and other sensitive tissues, and protects your organs. Wow! Good reasons for drinking the adequate amount of water daily!

Water aids in getting rid of waste in your body. Water helps you cleanse and detoxify, flushing out toxins from the body. A clean system is a healthy system!

Water helps you lose weight. Water is one of the best tools for weight loss; it's an appetite suppressant, and often when we think we're hungry, we're actually just thirsty. Being chronically dehydrated puts our system out of balance, causing us to binge and crave unhealthy foods. Water is the foundation to good health!

Water helps prevent clogging of arteries in the heart and the brain. Yet 90-95% of people are not drinking enough water and reaping the benefits. Stay on the prevention plan by staying hydrated. Water equals health, healing, and life!

Water supports the body's electromagnetic energy-system. Being dehydrated saps your energy and makes you tired; even mild dehydration effects your energy level. Dehydration can lead to fatigue, muscle weakness, dizziness, and other symptoms. So easy to energize your body with water!

Water helps cure headaches–often when we have headaches, it's simply a matter of not drinking enough water. There are lots of other causes of headaches of course, but dehydration is a common one.

Day 2

Pray and ask the Lord to speak to you. Read these verses out loud then answer the questions.
"Oh, give thanks to the Lord, for He is good! For His mercy endures forever. Let the redeemed of the Lord say so, whom He has redeemed from the hand of the enemy. Oh, that men would give thanks to the Lord for His goodness, and for His wonderful works to the children of men. For He satisfies the longing soul, and fills the hungry soul with goodness. There were those who dwelt in darkness and in the shadow of death, prisoners in misery and chains, because they rebelled against the words of God, and despised the counsel of the Most High. They fell down, and there was none to help. Then they cried out to the Lord in their trouble, and He saved them out of their distresses. He brought them out of darkness and the shadow of death, and broke their chains in pieces.
Oh, that men would give thanks to the Lord for His goodness, and for His wonderful works to the children of men! Whoever is wise will observe these things, and they will understand the lovingkindness of the Lord." (Psa. 107:1-2, 8-13, 43) "Death and life are in the power of the tongue, and those who love it will eat its fruit." (Prov. 18:21) "Do not grumble, as some of them did—and were killed by the destroying angel." (1 Cor. 10:10)

- **Why should you give thanks to the Lord?**
- **What does it mean to be redeemed?**
- **How does God satisfy you?**
- **What does He use to bring you life, and fill your soul with His goodness?**
- **If your heart is heavy, hurt, angry, bitter, or anxious, what should you do to satisfy your soul with good?**
- **How important is it to your soul to remember the goodness of God and that you are free, complete, righteous, and a new creation now with Christ?**
- **What things does giving thanks to God for His great work keep you from?**
- **Why is it wise to think and meditate on God's goodness toward you that He delivered you from the enemy?**
- **Is thanksgiving a matter of life and death?**
- **What happens to your perspective and soul when you give thanks?**
- **What happens to your perspective and soul when you complain?**
- **For what things in your life will you give words of thanksgiving, and bring life to them?**

AS YOU GO
As you go through your day, focus your mind on all the amazing blessings you receive by doing God's will and giving thanks in everything. Smile, shine God's glory, and give thanks to people for something at least 3x a day.

AFFIRMATION
Thank You, God, for all your amazing love and mercy and for delivering me from the hand of the enemy! I will give thanks and release life to every part of me!

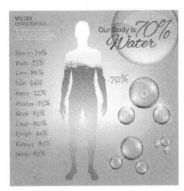

WATER TIPS

Water helps you have healthy skin, and drinking water can clear up your skin. Drinking the adequate amount of water helps keep the skin clear, glowing, and moist. It also delays the aging process. When you are dehydrated, the skin suffers. Water keeps you looking good!

Water helps you avoid digestive problems–our systems need a good amount of water to digest food properly. Often water can help cure stomach acid problems and, along with fiber, can cure constipation (often a result of dehydration). If you don't have a love relationship with water, begin one today!

Caffeine is a diuretic, so you need to drink more water for the extra fluid you lose. F. Batmanghelidj, MD shares testimony of how after a man stopped all caffeine for a week, drank ten glasses of water, and added ½ teaspoon of unrefined sea salt, he was cured. Not only was his blood pressure much lower, but he was freed from headaches, lower back pain, his sinuses were cleared, and no constipation!

Drinking the adequate amount of water daily has been found to reduce the risk of colon cancer by 45%, reduce the risk of bladder cancer by 50%, and reduce the risk of breast cancer by 75%. Drink to live!

Drinking water maintains the viscosity of the blood, which helps prevent blood thickening and reduces risk of cardiovascular heart attacks and strokes. Along with blood, muscles, lungs, and the brain are mostly water. So many amazing benefits for staying hydrated!

Staying hydrated reduces the chances of bladder and urinary tract infections and helps prevent kidney stones. Water is such a blessing to your body!

Day 3

Pray and ask the Lord to speak to you. Read these verses out loud then answer the questions.

Now on his way to Jerusalem, Jesus traveled along the border between Samaria and Galilee. As he was going into a village, ten men who had leprosy met him. They stood at a distance and called out in a loud voice, "Jesus, Master, have mercy on us!" When he saw them, he said, "Go, show yourselves to the priests." And as they went, they were cleansed. One of them, when he saw he was healed, came back, praising God in a loud voice. He threw himself at Jesus' feet and thanked him–and he was a Samaritan. Jesus asked, "Were not all ten cleansed? Where are the other nine? Has no one returned to give praise to God except this foreigner?" Then he said to him, "Rise and go; your faith has made you well, (whole)." (Luke17:11-19) "Let us then approach God's throne of grace with confidence, so that we may receive mercy and find grace to help us in our time of need." (Heb. 4:16) "My God will supply all your needs according to His riches in glory in Christ Jesus. Now to our God and Father be the glory forever and ever. Amen." (Phil. 4:19-20)

- How did coming to Jesus for mercy help these hopeless lepers?
- How will coming to Jesus for mercy help you?
- What happened to the one who returned to give thanks?
- Why didn't the rest return to give thanks?
- Why do you think someone doesn't give thanks after you have blessed them in an exceptional way?
- How will giving thanks daily to God for delivering you from the hand of the enemy impact your heart, health, and relationships?
- What things do you need to bring with confidence to the throne of grace, and receive mercy and grace to help meet your needs?
- What are the extreme blessings God has given you for which you need to give Him thanks?
- How will giving thanks to God for supplying all your needs make you whole, healthy?
- God really does supply all, not some or most of your needs. How would thanking God for supplying your specific needs at home, work, etc. every day help you?
- Health is a big need! Do you believe and thank God daily for supplying your health needs?
- When you don't, what are you replacing thanksgiving with, and how is that affecting your life?
- How does Jesus see thanksgiving?

AS YOU GO
As you go through your day, focus your mind on all the amazing blessings you receive by doing God's will and giving thanks in everything. Smile, shine God's glory, and give thanks to people for something at least 3x a day.

AFFIRMATION
I come to Your throne of grace with confidence and receive mercy and find grace to help me in whatever I need. Thank You, God! Thank You for supplying all my needs through Christ!

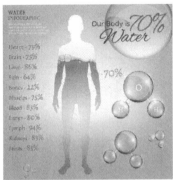

WATER TIPS

Drinking a couple of glasses of water right when you wake up is the perfect way to start your day off right! F. Batmanghelidj, MD says that the gradual rise in blood pressure is an indicator of a gradually establishing shortage of water in the body. We can avoid many sicknesses just by staying hydrated!

Water helps prevent the loss of memory as we age. It helps reduce the risk of Alzheimer's disease, multiple sclerosis, Parkinson's disease, and Lou Gehrig's disease.

Water is a brain booster–drink plenty of water before an important meeting, an exam, or any time when you need to enhance your mental abilities and concentration. Even a 2% drop in hydration can affect you physically and intellectually and slow down mental recall. There is evidence that lack of water can have more serious, long-term consequences such as neurological implications and depression.

Drinking an adequate amount of water daily is important for your overall good health because water aids in digestion, circulation, absorption, assimilation and even excretion. Every single system in your body is dependent on water. Prevent dehydration prevent disease!

When you are sick, you definitely need to drink many fluids. If you have a fever, vomiting, and diarrhea, all of these cause your body to lose water. When women breast-feed they will lose more water during that process and need to keep the water coming.

Water should be our first reaction to headaches, hunger between meals, digestion issues, bloating, vocal fatigue, muscle ache, and dry skin. Most of us are blessed to have the luxury of water on demand. As you drink, be aware of the gift you are giving yourself and all the amazing bodily-functions that the water is supporting.

Day 4

Pray and ask the Lord to speak to you. Read these verses out loud then answer the questions.
Some people came and told Jehoshaphat, "A vast army is coming against you from Edom, from the other side of the Dead Sea. Then Jehoshaphat prayed... "Lord, the God of our ancestors, are you not the God who is in heaven? You rule over all the kingdoms of the nations. Power and might are in your hand, and no one can withstand you. ... For we have no power to face this vast army that is attacking us. We do not know what to do, but our eyes are on you." Then Jahaziel said: "Listen, King Jehoshaphat and all who live in Judah and Jerusalem! This is what the Lord says to you: 'Do not be afraid or discouraged because of this vast army. For the battle is not yours, but God's. You will not have to fight this battle. Take up your positions; stand firm and see the deliverance the Lord will give you, Judah, and Jerusalem. Jehoshaphat stood and said, ... "Have faith in the Lord your God and you will be upheld; have faith in his prophets and you will be successful." Jehoshaphat appointed men to sing to the Lord and to praise him for the splendor of his holiness as they went out at the head of the army, saying: "Praise and give thanks to the Lord, for His mercy and lovingkindness endure forever." As they began to sing and praise, the Lord set ambushes against the people who were invading Judah, and they were defeated. When the men of Judah came to the place that overlooks the desert and looked toward the vast army, they saw only dead bodies lying on the ground; no one had escaped. (2 Chro. 20:2, 5-6, 12, 14-15, 17, 20-22, 24)

- Why do you think the lepers from day 3 and Jehoshaphat got results and won their battles?
- What do you need to realize in order to receive God's mercy?
- What did Jehoshaphat pray?
- What would happen if you prayed this way over your family, health, and other issues in your life?
- Who is in control of your battles, struggles?
- How will letting God control your life and battles impact your life?
- How did thanks and praise to God replace fear?
- How does praying from victory like they did change your perspective in prayer?
- What does that kind of prayer do to fear in your life?
- What did they do when they found out that the battle was God's and not theirs?
- If the battles in your life belong to the Lord, what should you do?
- How hard is it for you to give God total control of things, especially that are really challenging, and put your faith in His truth, love, and mercy and give thanks to Him?
- How are these verses helping you rethink God's will for you in Christ to rejoice always, pray continually, and give thanks in everything?
- Why is it important to keep reading the "AS YOU GO" even though it's the same every day?

AS YOU GO
As you go through your day, focus your mind on all the amazing blessings you receive by doing God's will and giving thanks in everything. Smile, shine God's glory, and give thanks to people for something at least 3x a day.

AFFIRMATION
I have no power apart from You, God, to overcome battles in my life. My eyes are on You. The battle is not mine, but Yours, God! I'm taking my position of praise and thanks to You for Your love and mercy and will see the deliverance the Lord!

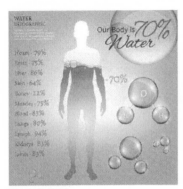

WATER TIPS
Staying hydrated helps solve constipation and indigestion problems. Water generates electrical and magnetic energy inside each and every cell of the body–it provides the power to live.

Comparative shortage of water first suppresses and eventually kills some aspects of the body. Signs of mild dehydration: thirst, loss of appetite, dry skin, darkened urine, dry mouth, fatigue, chills, and head rushes.

Water helps reverse addictive urges. We can keep ourselves out of so much health trouble by simply staying hydrated. Signs of moderate dehydration: increased heart rise, respiration, and body temperature, decreased sweating and urination, extreme fatigue, muscle cramps, headaches, nausea, and tingling of the limbs.

Signs of serious dehydration: muscle spasms, vomiting, racing pulse, shriveled skin, dim vision, painful urination, confusion, difficulty breathing, seizures, chest and abdominal pain, and unconsciousness. Dehydration is by far the most frequent constant stressor in the human body that raises blood pressure–in at least sixty million Americans, says F. Batmanghelidj, MD in His book, "You're Not Sick, You're Thirsty!"

Water your body. Think of a plant without water and how it wilts and dies. Just giving it water can spring it to life. Water is just as essential for our bodies because it is in every cell, tissue, and organ in your body. Water prevents DNA damage. Drinking water speeds up your metabolism.

Water increases the efficiency of red blood cells in the collecting oxygen in the lungs.

Day 5

Pray and ask the Lord to speak to you. Read these verses out loud then answer the questions.
"When my soul fainted within me, I remembered the Lord; and my prayer went up to You, into Your holy temple. "Those who regard worthless idols forsake their own Mercy. But I will sacrifice to You with the voice of thanksgiving; I will pay what I have vowed. Salvation is of the Lord." So the Lord spoke to the fish, and it vomited Jonah onto dry land." (Jonah 2:7-10) "Without faith it is impossible to please God, because anyone who comes to him must believe that he exists and that he rewards those who earnestly seek him." (Heb. 11:6) "Whoever calls on the name of the Lord shall be saved." (Rom. 10:13)

- **Jonah, who was in disobedience to God, was dying in the belly of a fish. What did He come to realize and receive from God?**
- **How does this story relate to what God said in day 2, to give thanks to the Lord for He is good, He has delivered you from the hand of the enemy?**
- **Why did God give the lepers, Jehoshaphat, and Jonah mercy and rescue them?**
- **How do you forsake (quit, leave, give up) mercy, this VALUABLE thing, and how do you receive it?**
- **What things have you done in your life that you think God can't undo and resurrect?**
- **What does God reward? How did Jonah enter God's holy temple and get rewarded by God?**
- **No matter where you are in life and all that's happened to you, how do these verses encourage you to come with faith in God's mercy to reward you?**
- **How can you put your faith in God right now and receive life for something that's dying in your life? (Relationship, health, finances, spiritual life, etc,)**
- **What are you learning about praying with thanks in the last 5 days, and how is your heart growing in gratitude toward God?**

AS YOU GO
As you go through your day focus your mind on all the amazing blessings you receive by doing God's will and giving thanks in everything. Smile, shine God's glory, and give thanks to people for something at least 3x a day.

AFFIRMATION:
I put my trust in You, God! I will sacrifice to You with the voice of thanksgiving. Salvation comes from You. I call on the name of the Lord for mercy and I will be saved!

GIVE THANKS
RELEASING GOD'S POWER TO BE WHOLE

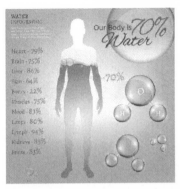

WATER TIPS

Water is a natural appetite suppressant and helps you to effortlessly lose weight! Dehydration is many times the cause of back pain. The bones of your vertebrae are supported by discs. And each disc is made up of water, so lacking water leads to back pain.

Water helps you in your exercising–being dehydrated can severely hamper your athletic activities, slowing you down and making it harder to lift weights. Dehydration causes cramping. Water, being a natural lubricant to your muscles and joints, makes you more flexible, less likely to experience sprained ankles, and less likely to be sore after working out.

Being dehydrated by just 2% impairs performance in tasks that require attention, psychomotor and immediate memory skills, as well as assessment of the subjective state. These are four ways dehydration affects your brain. Dehydration affects your mood. Dehydration reduces your cognitive and motor skills. Dehydration makes you more sensitive to pain. Dehydration affects your memory. The mind is a terrible thing to waste, drink up!

Dehydration will harm your skin. Drinking water is great for your skin. It helps to moisturize it, keep it soft, and removes wrinkles. Water to the body is absolutely vital for making the immune system more efficient in fighting infections and cancer cells.

People have been healed of asthma, allergies, diabetes, and degenerated lumbar spine from just simply drinking enough water daily! You need water to provide the means for nutrients to travel to your organs and tissues. Water also helps transport oxygen to your cells.

Day 6

Pray and ask the Lord to speak to you. Read these verses out loud then answer the questions.

"Jesus said to her, "I am the Resurrection and the Life. Whoever believes in (adheres to, trusts in, relies on) Me [as Savior] will live even if he dies; and everyone who lives and believes in Me [as Savior] will never die. Do you believe this?"

Jesus said to her, "Did I not say to you that if you would believe you would see the glory of God?" Then they took away the stone from the place where the dead man was lying. And Jesus lifted up His eyes and said, "Father, I thank You that You have heard Me. And I know that You always hear Me, but because of the people who are standing by I said this, that they may believe that You sent Me." Now when He had said these things, He cried with a loud voice, "Lazarus, come forth!" And he who had died came out bound hand and foot with grave clothes, and his face was wrapped with a cloth. Jesus said to them, "Loose him, and let him go." (John 11:25-26, 40-44) "For with the heart one believes unto righteousness, and with the mouth confession is made unto salvation." (Rom. 10:10) "Humble yourselves under the mighty hand of God, so that He may exalt you [to a place of honor in His service] at the appropriate time, casting all your cares [all your anxieties, all your worries, and all your concerns, once and for all] on Him, for He cares about you [with deepest affection, and watches over you very carefully]." (1 Pet. 5:6-7)

"Truly, truly, I say to you, he who believes in Me, the works that I do, he will do also; and greater works than these he will do; because I go to the Father. Whatever you ask in My name, that will I do, so that the Father may be glorified in the Son. If you ask Me anything in My name, I will do it." (John 14:12-14) "We walk by faith, not by sight." (2 Cor. 5:7)

- Why didn't the woman believe Jesus would raise her brother from the dead and give him life right now?
- What did Jesus say she would see if she believed his words, that He is the Resurrection and Life in her present situation?
- How will you see God's glory and receive life and resurrection from Jesus by believing His words right now, and remove your darkness, pain, addiction, bitterness, hurt, and even sickness?
- What did the lepers, Jehoshaphat, Jonah, and Jesus believe about the Father?
- If you believe someone is good, willing, and has the ability to help you, do you believe that they will help you?
- What's something for which you can begin giving God thanks, and believing He is good and will help you to receive good, impossible things?
- How did the lepers, Jehoshaphat, Jonah, and Jesus overcome the impossible?
- How did they overcome anxiety, fear, and worry, and receive the blessing from God when going through difficulty?
- What will happen to your impossible situations if you begin humbling yourself to God and believing His word, rather than what you see or hear?
- How did Jesus pray?

- Could receiving the impossible, salvation (healing, deliverance, freedom, protection, wholeness), really be as easy as believing with your heart in God's love and mercy toward you and confessing His words of truth with your mouth?

- Once you've received Jesus as Your Savior, you've died with Christ and now you've been made alive, because He now lives in you! Since Jesus is now you're life and everything in your life is in His care, what things can you begin giving to Him to care for?

- God is the greatest Giver! He gave you His own Son! You are a receiver. How can you be a good receiver?

- Why should it be easy to bless His name and give Him thanks in all your circumstances if you've already received salvation?

- How will walking by faith in what God's word says, rather than what you see, keep you blessing His name at all times?

- How aware are you of God's presence with you at ALL times? Are you casting ALL your cares on Him and living free from anxiety?

AS YOU GO

As you go through your day, focus your mind on all the MANY amazing blessings you've received through God's love and mercy, and how grateful you are for Jesus. Smile, shine God's glory, and give thanks to people for something at least 3x a day.

AFFIRMATION

I believe that Jesus, who is the Resurrection and Life, lives in me and cares for all my needs! I live by faith, not sight, and confess Him as Lord of my life daily by giving Him thanks in everything!

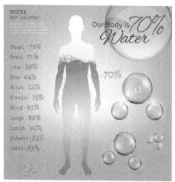

WATER TIPS

Drinking water helps maintain blood pressure. A lack of water can cause blood to become thicker, increasing blood pressure. Water delivers oxygen throughout the body. Blood is more than 80 percent water, and blood carries oxygen to different parts of the body. Healthy blood, healthy body; drink to live!

Water helps reduce stress, anxiety, and depression. Your body will work better in every way when properly hydrated. Therefore you're more likely to feel better about yourself!

Healthy people stay hydrated everyday. Keep your urine clear. That shows you are properly hydrated. When your urine is a dark yellow or has an odor, you are definitely dehydrated. Note: riboflavin, a B vitamin, will make your urine bright yellow when you take dietary supplements that contain large amounts of riboflavin. Certain medications can change the color of urine as well.

Water restores normal sleep rhythms. Water gives luster and shine to the eyes. Water helps prevent glaucoma.

Your body needs more water when you are in hot climates, more physically active, running a fever or have diarrhea or vomiting.

Water normalizes the blood-manufacturing systems in the bone marrow–it helps prevent leukemia and lymphoma.

GIVE THANKS
RELEASING GOD'S POWER TO BE WHOLE

Day 7

Pray and ask the Lord to speak to you. Read these verses out loud then answer the questions.
"Make a joyful shout to the Lord, all you lands! Serve the Lord with gladness; come before His presence with singing. Know that the Lord, He is God; it is He who has made us, and not we ourselves; we are His people and the sheep of His pasture. Enter into His gates with thanksgiving, and into His courts with praise. Be thankful to Him, and bless His name. For the Lord is good; His mercy is everlasting, and His truth endures to all generations." (Psa. 100)
"Do not be anxious about anything, but in every situation, by prayer and petition, with thanksgiving, present your requests to God. And the peace of God, which transcends all understanding, will guard your hearts and your minds in Christ Jesus. Finally, brothers and sisters, whatever is true, noble, right, pure, lovely, of a good report, admirable–if anything is excellent or praiseworthy–think about such things." (Phil. 4:6-8) "Whoever dwells in the shelter of the Most High will rest in the shadow of the Almighty, I will say of the Lord, "He is my refuge and my fortress, my God, in whom I trust. Because you have made the Lord, who is my refuge, Even the Most High, your dwelling place, no evil shall befall you, Nor shall any plague come near your dwelling. With long life I will satisfy him, and show him My salvation." (Psa. 91:1-2, 9-10) "I am the vine; you are the branches. If you remain in me and I in you, you will bear much fruit; apart from me you can do nothing." (John 15:5) "Above all else, guard your heart, for everything you do flows from it." (Prov. 4:23) "A heart at peace gives life to the body." (Prov. 14:30) "God will meet all your needs according to the riches of his glory in Christ Jesus." (Phil. 4:19)

- How do you enter God's presence (gates) of love, joy, mercy, and peace to meet with Him and hear His voice?
- What are you to NEVER do?
- What are you to do in EVERY situation?
- Why is God COMMANDING you to guard your heart and pray with thanks?
- How do you easily guard your heart?
- Your heart is the place of gratitude, praise, and worship to God, so what is God trying to keep you from? Why?
- What does praying with thanksgiving do to your anxious thoughts and feelings and what other changes are you experiencing through thanksgiving?
- What do you remember from 1 Thess. 5 in Day 1 that God's peace does for you?
- How much peace does God supply for you when you enter His holy presence by praying with thanksgiving?
- If a heart at peace gives you health (life) to your whole body, what does a heart of fear and anxiety cause to happen to your body?
- What does worrying say you believe about God?
- What does giving thanks say you believe about God?
- God wants your thoughts VERY positive all the time. Why?
- How does giving thanks to God relate to abiding/dwelling in Him?

- What is the secret way of speaking to abide in Him and receive a long satisfied life, one of love, joy, and peace, and see God's healing and restoring work in your life?
- Where do you feel dissatisfied with your life? What will bring satisfaction to that or those areas?
- Will you take the challenge of giving thanks to God in those areas to begin finding satisfaction?
- Abiding and remaining in thanksgiving to God daily is a hundred percent guarantee to God's work of bearing fruit. How much fruit? What kind of fruit? What areas of your life are you not experiencing fruit? Can you give it to Him right now?

Pray over something that concerns you with thanksgiving. God's peace is an AMAZING AND POWERFUL GIFT! Then thank God for His peace!

AS YOU GO

As you go through your day, focus your mind on all the MANY amazing blessings you've received through God's love and mercy and how grateful you are for Jesus. Smile, shine God's glory, and give thanks to people for something at least 3x a day.

AFFIRMATION:

I enter God's presence with thanks and live in His peace that goes beyond understanding! I have nothing to worry about in God's presence! I'm fully protected and given a long, satisfied, healthy life in God's presence!

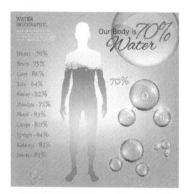

WATER TIPS

All the cell and organ functions that make up our entire anatomy and physiology depend on water for their functioning. Water dilutes the blood and prevents it from clotting during circulation.

Do not drink water during meals as it hampers the digestion by reducing the concentration of gastric juices that aids the process of digestion. Drink two glasses of water after waking up. This will help to activate the internal organs. Drink one glass of water 30 minutes before meals. This helps in digestion. Drink one glass of water before taking a bath. This helps to lower your blood pressure. Drink one glass of water before bedtime. This helps to avoid stroke or heart attack. Drink one glass of water before workouts. This helps to arm you against dehydration during an indoor or outdoor workout. Drink water after workouts. This helps to replace fluids lost by sweating and physical labor.

Back pain can be caused by dehydration when the body rations water away from the joints. Less lubrication equals greater friction and that can cause joint, knee, and back pain, potentially leading to injuries and arthritis.

Water makes up more than two thirds of human body weight, and without water, we would die in a few days. The human brain is made up of 95% water, blood is 82%, and lungs 90%. A mere 2% drop in our body's water supply can trigger signs of dehydration: fuzzy short-term memory, trouble with basic math, and difficulty focusing on smaller print, such as a computer screen. (Are you having trouble reading this? Drink up!) Mild dehydration is also one of the most common causes of daytime fatigue. An estimated seventy-five percent of Americans have mild, chronic dehydration. What a scary statistic for a developed country where water is readily available.

Day 8

Welcome to your smoothie week! Let food be your medicine! Don't forget to keep drinking your eight glasses of water also. Everything counts so don't worry about not getting it all right just keep moving forward with thanksgiving and things will get better and changes will happen.

Pray and ask the Lord to speak to you. Read these verses out loud then answer the questions.
"I will be merciful to their unrighteousness, and their sins and their lawless deeds I will remember no more." (Heb. 8:12) "I will praise You, O Lord, with my whole heart; I will tell of all Your marvelous works. I will be glad and rejoice in You; I will sing praise to Your name, O Most High." (Psa. 9:1-2) "Praise be to the God and Father of our Lord Jesus Christ! In His great mercy he has given us new birth into a living hope through the resurrection of Jesus Christ from the dead, and into an inheritance that can never perish, spoil or fade. This inheritance is kept in heaven for you, who through faith are shielded by God's power... In all this you greatly rejoice, though now for a little while you may have had to suffer grief in all kinds of trials. These have come so that the proven genuineness of your faith–of greater worth than gold." (1 Pet. 1:3-7) "As for you, you were dead in your transgressions and sins. But because of His great love for us, God, who is rich in mercy, made us alive with Christ even when we were dead in transgressions–it is by grace you have been saved. And God raised us up with Christ and seated us with him in the heavenly realms in Christ Jesus. For it is by grace you have been saved, through faith–and this is not from yourselves, it is the gift of God. (Eph. 2:1,4-6,8) "Count yourselves dead to sin but alive to God in Christ Jesus" (Rom. 6:11) "Thanks be to God for His indescribable gift!" (2 Cor. 9:15) "Through the Lord's mercies we are not consumed, because His compassions fail not. They are new every morning; great is Your faithfulness." (Lam. 3:22-24)

- **How does rejoicing in God's rich mercy change the way you see Him, yourself, and others?**
- **What GOOD work has God done for you through Christ that will make you praise Him with your whole heart?**
- **If you received a billion dollars and you never had to worry about money again, your response would be overflowing with joy! How do you respond daily to God for His rich mercy that covers over all your sins and sicknesses everyday?**
- **What was your condition before receiving God's mercy?**

GIVE THANKS
RELEASING GOD'S POWER TO BE WHOLE

- How did God's AMAZING grace and RICH mercy transform your condition, your identity, position, and life?
- Why should you GREATLY rejoice when going through a trial?
- How valuable is your faith in God's indescribable gift of Jesus?
- "Saved" is the Greek word "sozo" meaning "to be whole-physically, mentally and spiritually." How are you saved, made whole?
- What does putting your faith in God's words of truth do for you?
- What's an area of your life you need to be saved: physically, mentally, or spiritually?
- Remember in 1 Thess. 5 from Day 1 that said how God was faithful and He will do it, sanctify you completely through His peace, and make you whole? How does God make you whole, save you?

AS YOU GO

As you go through your day, focus your mind on all the MANY amazing blessings you've received through God's love and mercy and how grateful you are for Jesus. Smile, shine God's glory, and give thanks to people for something at least 4x a day.

AFFIRMATION:

Thanks be to God for His indescribable gift of mercy through Jesus! I live by grace through faith and give thanks in everything, and am shielded by God's power and made whole: spirit, soul, and body!

LIVING FOOD VERSES DEAD FOOD

"Death and life are in the power of the tongue, and those who love it and indulge it will eat its fruit and bear the consequences of their words." "The word of God is living and powerful." (Prov. 18:21; Heb. 4:12)

An excellent movie to watch on healthy eating that will significantly encourage you is called Forks Over Knives. You can watch a preview on YouTube. Forks Over Knives is on Netflix.

We should eat mostly living food, which consists of raw fruits, vegetables, grains, nuts and seeds. Our bodies are living organism comprised of living cells. The good news is that when we feed our bodies what they need, we don't crave the bad stuff. In the same way, when we feed our soul life by giving thanks in everything, we don't crave what will kill us.

Living food has not had its life force (enzymes) destroyed by heat. Processed sugar causes MANY diseases to our body. Living foods will make you feel better and look better!

All food that is cooked is dead food, and can't properly nourish the living cells. Raw and live foods nourish and improve the body's inner environment. Raw and live foods enable the body to dislodge and expel accumulated wastes. Putting God's word in your mouth removes the toxic emotions and thoughts that kill us!

Enzymes also help speed healing after surgery and chemotherapy, fight inflammation, and help boost our immune system as well as many other benefits. God's words of life heals and delivers us! (Psa. 107:20)

Enzymes found in living food play a crucial role in aiding our bodies in the process of proper digestion, elimination, and absorption of vital nutrients found in living food. Yes, and life and godliness are found in Jesus, the Word. (1 Pet. 1:2-4)

Dr. Edward Howell, pioneer of Enzyme Therapy said, "Enzymes are substances that make life possible... Without enzymes, no activity at all would take place." "He who has the Son has life; he who does not have the Son of God does not have life." (1 John 5:12)

Day 9

Pray and ask the Lord to speak to you. Read these verses out loud then answer the questions.
"Praise the Lord! He has heard my cry for mercy. The Lord is my strength and shield. I trust him with all my heart. He helps me, and my heart is filled with joy. I burst out in songs of thanksgiving." (Psa. 28:6-7)
"But you are a chosen generation, a royal priesthood, a holy nation, His own special people, that you may proclaim the praises of Him who called you out of darkness into His marvelous light; who once were not a people but are now the people of God, who had not obtained mercy but now have obtained mercy." (Pet. 2:9-10)

"The Helper, the Holy Spirit, whom the Father will send in My name, He will teach you all things... Peace I leave with you, My peace I give to you; not as the world gives do I give to you. Let not your heart be troubled, neither let it be afraid." (John 14:26-27)

"God is our refuge and strength, a very present help in trouble. Therefore we will not fear." (Psa. 46:1-2a)

"Fear not, for I am with you; be not dismayed, for I am your God. I will strengthen you, Yes, I will help you, I will uphold you with My righteous right hand." (Isa. 41:10)

"The Lord is my light and my salvation; whom shall I fear? The Lord is the strength of my life; of whom shall I be afraid?" (Psa. 27:1)

- **If it's true and God is merciful and provides you with physical, mental, and emotional strength, protection from the enemy, and help for ALL your needs, what should this good news cause you to be and do every day?**
- **What has God called you out of, and what has He called you into?**
- **Are you living in who you are in Christ, full of praise to God for His wonderful work of deliverance through His mercy?**
- **How does the peace that God has given you empower you to overcome fear?**
- **Why do you look for peace if you have already been given it?**

- How can you live daily in the peace of God?
- In the midst of struggle, how can God's way of giving thanks help you and teach you a new way that's fruitful?
- Jesus is with you always and is very present to help you. How do you see Him helping you in your relationships and health?
- How does giving thanks in everything strengthen you in the Lord? How will these verses for today encourage you and help you to choose thanksgiving?
- Why does God keep telling us to not fear, to not let our heart be troubled?
- Pray and thank the Holy Spirit for being your helper in every area of your life.
- Thank Him for helping you and giving you power to be a blessing in your relationships, finances, ministry, and health. Thank Him for teaching you how to be an excellent spouse, friend, parent, encourager, etc... Thank Him for teaching you how to live a healthy lifestyle and helping you make any changes you need to make.
- The Bible says in James 4:3 that you have not because you fail to ask. How does asking God daily to help you and teach you things cause you not to lack in these areas?

AS YOU GO

As you go through your day, focus your mind on all the MANY amazing blessings you've received through God's love and mercy, and how grateful you are for Jesus. Smile, shine God's glory, and give thanks to people for something at least 4x a day.

AFFIRMATION:

Peace You gave to me; therefore I will not let my heart be troubled, neither will I let it be afraid. Thank You for being with me and being my God. Thank You for strengthening and helping me more everyday and for upholding me with Your righteous right hand.

LIVING FOOD VERSES DEAD FOOD

"Death and life are in the power of the tongue, and those who love it and indulge it will eat its fruit and bear the consequences of their words." "The word of God is living and powerful." (Prov. 18:21; Heb. 4:12)

Neither vitamins, minerals, or hormones can do any work without enzymes. Aim for eating 50-80% living food daily. Bananas contain high levels of fructooligosaccharide, which promote calcium absorption and nourish healthy bacteria in the colon that manufactures vitamins and digestive enzymes which boost the body's overall ability to absorb nutrients.

Dr. Francis Pottenger did an experiment in which he fed 900 cats the same foods for nine years. However, half of the cats ate their food raw and the other half ate their food cooked. The cats that ate their food raw over the nine years never suffered any physical problem. But he observed that the cats that ate the cooked food developed the same physical problems from which many people in civilized societies suffer, and the longer the cats ate the dead/cooked food, the earlier the cats experienced sickness.

Raw fed cats' internal organs show full development and normal function. Over their life spans, they prove resistant to infections, to fleas, and to various other parasites, and show no signs of allergies. In general, they are gregarious, friendly, and predictable in their behavior patterns, and when thrown or dropped as much as six feet to test their coordination, they always land on their feet and come back for more play. These cats reproduce one homogeneous generation after another. Miscarriages are rare, and the litters average five kittens with the mother cat nursing her young without difficulty.

All occur commonly in Cooked-meat-fed, cats. The bones are abnormally brittle and subject to fracture, heart problems; nearsightedness and farsightedness; under activity of the thyroid or inflammation of the thyroid gland; infections of the kidney, of the liver, of the testes, of the ovaries, and of the bladder; arthritis and inflammation of the joints; inflammation of the nervous system with paralysis and meningitis.

The third generation of cats are much more irritability. Some females are even dangerous to handle because of their proclivity for biting and scratching. Their lungs show hyperemia, while the most deficient show bronchitis and pneumonitis. Their newborns are very physiologically bankrupt so much that none survive beyond the sixth month of life.

"Do not work for food that spoils, but for food that endures to eternal life, which the Son of Man will give you. Then Jesus declared, 'I am the bread of life. Whoever comes to me will never go hungry, and whoever believes in me will never be thirsty." John 6:27,35

Day 10

Pray and ask the Lord to speak to you. Read these verses out loud then answer the questions.
"Ask, and it will be given to you; seek, and you will find; knock, and it will be opened to you. For everyone who asks receives, and he who seeks finds, and to him who knocks it will be opened. Or what man is there among you who, if his son asks for bread, will give him a stone? Or if he asks for a fish, will he give him a serpent? If you then, being evil, know how to give good gifts to your children, how much more will your Father who is in heaven give good things to those who ask Him!" (Matt. 7:7-11)

"As for me, I will always have hope; I will praise you more and more." (Ps. 71:14)

"As evening approached, the disciples came to him and said, "This is a remote place, and it's already getting late. Send the crowds away, so they can go to the villages and buy themselves some food." Jesus replied, "They do not need to go away. You give them something to eat." "We have here only five loaves of bread and two fish," they answered. "Bring them here to me," he said. And he directed the people to sit down on the grass. Taking the five loaves and the two fish and looking up to heaven, he gave thanks and broke the loaves. Then he gave them to the disciples, and the disciples gave them to the people. They all ate and were satisfied, and the disciples picked up twelve basketfuls of broken pieces that were left over. The number of those who ate was about five thousand men, besides women and children." (Matt. 14:15-21)

"Therefore I tell you, whatever you ask for in prayer, believe that you have received it, and it will be yours." (Mark 11:24)

- **Do you think that giving thanks has anything to do with trusting the Lord with all your heart?**
- **Why did Jesus pray with thanks?**
- **How long was His prayer?**
- **What do you suppose Jesus knew about the Father's love by asking for the boy's lunch and simply praying with thanks?**
- **Are you finding more and more things to praise and thank God for or less and less?**

- When you pray, do you pray in faith with thanks for the results, or pray but don't expect to see anything happen?
- What will give you the same kind of faith in the Father's love as Jesus when you pray?
- How did one person's believing prayer impact many people?
- How can you begin praying in faith with thanks about impossibilities and impact many people around you at home, work, church, and neighborhood?
- Jesus sees and believes totally different than the disciples. Why?
- How do you see yourself: like Jesus or the disciples when there's an impossible situation?
- What did the lepers, Jehoshaphat, Jonah, and Jesus all believe about the Father's love?
- What do you remember about God's mercy?
- Pray right now for God's mercy over the impossible things in your life and thank the Father for showing His mercy! He's rich in mercy!

AS YOU GO
As you go through your day, focus your mind on all the MANY amazing blessings you've received through God's love and mercy, and how grateful you are for Jesus. Smile, shine God's glory, and give thanks to people for something at least 4x a day.

AFFIRMATION:
Whatever I ask for in prayer, I believe that I have received it and thank the Father for it and it will be mine. I believe because God says to ask and I will receive, not might receive. My Father loves to give me good things!

LIVING FOOD VERSES DEAD FOOD
"Death and life are in the power of the tongue, and those who love it and indulge it will eat its fruit and bear the consequences of their words." "The word of God is living and powerful." (Prov. 18:21; Heb. 4:12)

Those who live on living foods are better rested and better rested during sleep in less time. The worst of dead foods are refined flour and added sugar–they may actually suck stored vitamins out of your body as your system tries to metabolize them.

Those who eat mostly living foods are more alert and think clearer, sharper, and more logically.

Live food eaters feel better and have more energy and stamina.

The high amounts of potassium in bananas can restock electrolytes that are easily depleted when suffering from diarrhea–potassium being an important electrolyte itself.

Those who rely upon living foods become more active and precise in their motions and actions, as well as their thoughts. Hence they perform much better and with more competence.

Food is fuel and dead food is a very low-grade fuel, which is not capable of adequately nourishing our living bodies, comprised of living cells.

Best of all, live food eaters become virtually sickness free! Live food eaters are less subject to stresses and nervous tensions. Cooking destroys vitamins in food rather quickly.

"Listen carefully to Me, and eat what is good, and let your soul delight itself in abundance. Incline your ear, and come to Me. Hear, and your soul shall live." (Isa. 55:2-3) When you listen to God's word, you are eating good food and receiving an abundance of life!

GIVE THANKS
RELEASING GOD'S POWER TO BE WHOLE

Day 11

Pray and ask the Lord to speak to you. Read these verses out loud then answer the questions.
"He also brought me up out of a horrible pit, out of the miry clay, and set my feet upon a rock, and established my steps. He has put a new song in my mouth–Praise to our God; many will see it and fear, and will trust in the Lord. Blessed is that man who makes the Lord his trust, and has not turned to the proud or to the followers of lies. O Lord my God, many are the great works You have done, and Your thoughts toward us. No one can compare with You! If I were to speak and tell of them, there would be too many to number. I am happy to do Your will, O my God. Your Law is within my heart. I have told the good news about what is right and good with many people. You know I will not close my lips, O Lord. I have not hidden what is right and good with You in my heart. I have spoken about how faithful You are and about Your saving power. I have not hidden Your loving-kindness and Your truth." (Psa. 40:2-5, 8-10)

"I will bless the Lord at all times; His praise shall continually be in my mouth. My soul shall make its boast in the Lord... Oh, magnify the Lord with me, and let us exalt His name together. I sought the Lord, and He heard me, and delivered me from all my fears. The angel of the Lord encamps all around those who fear Him, and delivers them. Oh, taste and see that the Lord is good; blessed is the man who trusts in Him! The young lions lack and suffer hunger; but those who seek the Lord shall not lack any good thing. Many are the afflictions of the righteous, but the Lord delivers him out of them all." (Psa. 34:1-4, 6-8, 10, 19)

- **When God took you out of that horrible pit of sin through Jesus, what did He put in your mouth?**
- **Why?**
- **Why are you blessed when you trust in the Lord and praise Him?**
- **Many are the great works God has done for you in Christ; too many to number! Can you name 10 of them? Could you name 10 new ones everyday?**
- **What is God's will for your heart and mouth? How happy are you doing God's will daily?**
- **What are the benefits of blessing the Lord at all times and continually praising Him with your mouth?**
- **How did Jehoshaphat and Jonah trust in the Lord and experience their deliverance?**
- **How will you trust in the Lord and experience deliverance, freedom from afflictions, fear, oppression, or any other difficulty?**
- **Remember, there's power for life and death in your words. What do these verses tell you about your mouth?**
- **What will you lack when you trust the Lord and bless Him, giving Him thanks in all your circumstances?**
- **How can you pray and trust the Lord right now for an area in your life you feel like you are lacking?**
- **What happens to all your fears when you praise the Lord?**

AS YOU GO

As you go through your day, focus your mind on all the MANY amazing blessings you've received through God's love and mercy, and how grateful you are for Jesus. Smile, shine God's glory and give thanks to people for something at least 4x a day.

AFFIRMATION:

I will bless the Lord at all times; His praise shall continually be in my mouth and I will lack no good thing! I put my trust in the Lord and praise Him and He delivers me from all my fears! I speak of His great works He's done for me all day long!

LIVING FOOD VERSES DEAD FOOD

"Death and life are in the power of the tongue, and those who love it and indulge it will eat its fruit and bear the consequences of their words." "The word of God is living and powerful." (Prov. 18:21; Heb. 4:12)

Heated fats, oils, are especially damaging because they are altered to form acroleins, free radicals, other mutagens and carcinogens as confirmed in the publication, "Diet, Nutrition and Cancer."

Cooked foods not only take longer to digest, but often prove to be indigestible and unassailable as in the case of heated proteins.

Cooked foods quickly ferment and putrefy in the intestinal tract while living foods are almost totally absorbed before they're oxidized enough for yeast and bacterial ferments and putrefaction.

The average conventional eater has about two pounds of intestinal bacteria whereas living food eaters have only a few ounces.

About 20% of the feces of cooked food eaters is dead bacteria, whereas living food eaters give off only a fraction as much dead bacteria.

The chemical additives, preservatives, and man-made fats are also toxic to your system, and they are stored as plaque, which clogs your arteries.

Jesus answered, "It is written: 'Man shall not live on bread alone, but on every word that comes from the mouth of God." Taste and see that the Lord is good; blessed is the one who takes refuge in him." (Matt. 4:4; Psa. 34:8)

Day 12

Pray and ask the Lord to speak to you. Read these verses out loud then answer the questions.
"Do not be foolish, but understand what the Lord's will is. Do not get drunk on wine, which leads to debauchery. Instead, be filled with the Spirit, speaking to one another with psalms, hymns, and songs from the Spirit. Sing and make music from your heart to the Lord, always giving thanks to God the Father for everything, in the name of our Lord Jesus Christ." (Eph. 5:17-20)

"For God has not given us a spirit of fear, but of power and of love and of a sound mind." (2 Tim. 1:7)

"The fruit of the Spirit is love, joy, peace, patience, kindness, goodness, faithfulness, gentleness, self-control." (Gal. 5:22-23)

"There is no fear in love. But perfect love drives out fear, because fear has to do with punishment. The one who fears is not made perfect in love." (1 John 4:18)

- **What is the Lord's will?**
- **What will you be if you don't do the Lord's will?**
- **What good things will you enjoy by being filled with God's Spirit?**
- **What kind of qualities in others do you most admire? Why?**
- **Are the qualities that you most admire the fruit of God's Spirit?**
- **What do your words have to do with being filled with His Spirit?**
- **Words have power and fear brings death, but love brings life. What words will fill you with the power, love, and sound mind of God's Spirit?**
- **What do your words have to do with being filled with fear?**
- **What kinds of words fill you with fear?**
- **Are your words filled with love or fear?**
- **Where does fear come from?**
- **What do your thoughts, emotions, and attitude become like if you are filled with fear?**
- **What do your thoughts, emotions (heart), and attitude become like if you are filled with God's Spirit?**
- **How much fear is in love?**
- **What does love do to fear?**
- **Pray with thanks right now for God's love. Did you experience any fear while you were praying?**
- **When you feel fear, how hard would it be to simply stop and pray with thanks to God for His love?**
- **Jesus took all your judgment, punishment, and sin on the cross, so that you can live in the Father's love and be free from fear! God wants you to overcome fear by giving thanks in everything. How can remembering this extremely good news daily of God's way of escape through focusing on His love make it easy for you to give thanks always in everything, even hard situations?**

AS YOU GO
As you go through your day, focus your mind on all the MANY amazing blessings you've received through God's love and mercy, and how grateful you are for Jesus. Smile, shine God's glory, and give thanks to people for something at least 4x a day.

AFFIRMATION:
I give thanks always for everything and have the power, love, and sound mind of the Holy Spirit! I am filled with God's love by simply thanking and praising Him for His love. Fear is always quickly removed when I focus on God's love!

LIVING FOOD VERSES DEAD FOOD
"Death and life are in the power of the tongue, and those who love it and indulge it will eat its fruit and bear the consequences of their words." "The word of God is living and powerful." (Prov. 18:21; Heb. 4:12)

When your food is processed and preserved by the addition of refined flour, salt, sugar and chemicals, it literally sucks the life (vitamins, minerals and enzymes) out of your body, as it tries to digest and metabolize it.

There are no usable nutrients left, so you are under nourished. Your body craves more nutrients, so you end up overeating empty calories and becoming malnourished at the same time.

Everything you put in your mouth has the potential to make you healthy or sick.

At about 107 degrees, the enzymes that give life in raw plant foods start to die, and by about 122 degrees, all enzymes have been destroyed and living food becomes dead food.

When you are feeding your body with living food, you are feeding your body properly and will experience good health!

Life begets life! Dead food cannot properly sustain life! Dead food causes physical breakdown and ultimately sickness and an untimely and unnecessarily early death.

"How sweet are your words to my taste, sweeter than honey to my mouth! They are more precious than gold, than much pure gold; they are sweeter than honey, than honey from the honeycomb." (Psa. 119:103; 19:7-10)

Day 13

Pray and ask the Lord to speak to you. Read these verses out loud then answer the questions.
"But mark this: There will be terrible times in the last days. Men will be lovers of themselves...
unthankful, unholy, unloving, unforgiving, ... men of corrupt minds. (2 Tim. 3:1-2, 8)

"Although they knew God, they did not glorify Him as God, nor were thankful, but became futile in
their thoughts, and their foolish hearts were darkened." (Rom. 1:21)

"Self-seeking and envy are earthly, sensual, demonic. For where envy and self-seeking exist, confusion
and every evil thing are there. But the wisdom that is from above is first pure, then peaceable, gentle,
willing to yield, full of mercy and good fruits, without partiality and without hypocrisy. (James 3:14-17)
"Do not conform to the pattern of this world, but be transformed by the renewing of your mind. Then
you will be able to test and approve what God's will is—his good, pleasing and perfect will." (Rom.
12:2) "Do nothing out of selfish ambition or vain conceit. Rather, in humility value others above
yourselves, not looking to your own interests but each of you to the interests of the others... Do
everything without grumbling or arguing, so that you may become blameless and pure, "children of God
without fault in a warped and crooked generation." Then you will shine among them like stars in the
sky." (Phil. 2:3-4, 14-15)

- **What happens to your mind when you are unthankful, unloving, and unforgiving?**
- **What benefits in relationships do you experience by giving thanks, loving others, and
  forgiving?**
- **If you glorify God and give Him thanks, what will your mind and heart not become?**
- **What are synonyms and antonyms for futile?**
- **What words can you speak to have a fruitful, effective, and successful mind?**
- **What will renewing your mind with God's word and way do to you?**
- **Describe God's good, pleasing, and perfect will that you will experience by renewing your
  mind.**
- **Instead of grumbling, what words can you speak that will make you pure and shine like
  stars in the sky?**
- **How important is it for you to give thanks daily to God?**
- **How will giving thanks make you a better person?**
- **What kind of words lead to confusion and every evil thing?**
- **What kind of words lead to a sound mind and every good thing?**
- **How can you be more focused on others and their needs in conversations and less focused
  on you?**
- **What areas of your life will benefit from a humble attitude and giving thanks?**

GIVE THANKS
RELEASING GOD'S POWER TO BE WHOLE

AS YOU GO
As you go through your day, focus your mind on all the MANY amazing blessings you've received through God's love and mercy, and how grateful you are for Jesus. Smile, shine God's glory, and give thanks to people for something at least 4x a day.

AFFIRMATION:
I do nothing out of selfish ambition, but do everything with thanksgiving, and become pure and shine like stars in the sky. I glorify God and give Him thanks and have a successful mind.

LIVING FOOD VERSES DEAD FOOD
"Death and life are in the power of the tongue, and those who love it and indulge it will eat its fruit and bear the consequences of their words." "The word of God is living and powerful." (Prov. 18:21; Heb. 4:12)

Dead foods are the opposite of living. They are living foods that have fallen into human hands and have been altered in every imaginable way, making them last as long as possible at room temperature and to be as addictive as possible to the consumer.

There is a deadly, sludgy substance that is toxic to our bodies. That sludgy substance–which is called "hydrogenated" or "partially hydrogenated" oil–is a common ingredient in the American diet and is present in most processed foods.

Considerable amounts of sugar, which is called "dextrose," "corn syrup," "fructose," "glucose," and generally any other food ending in "ose" are added, doing much damage to our bodies!

When you eat living foods, the enzymes in their pristine state interact with your digestive enzymes. The other natural ingredients God put in them–vitamins, minerals, phytonutrients, antioxidants, fiber, and more–flow into your system in their natural state. These living foods were created for our digestive systems, bloodstream, and organs.

Dead foods hit our bodies like a foreign intruder. Chemicals, including preservatives, food additives, bleaching agents, and so on, place a strain on the liver. Eating cooked food prevents the immune system from working on what is really important in keeping us superbly healthy and young in body, mind, and soul.

Cooked foods cannot create true health because they are missing some very vital elements needed by the body for its optimal functioning; things like enzymes, oxygen, hormones, phytochemicals, bio-electrical energy and life-force.

"Do not work for food that spoils, but for food that endures to eternal life, which the Son of Man will give you. Then Jesus declared, "I am the bread of life. Whoever comes to me will never go hungry, and whoever believes in me will never be thirsty." (John 6:27, 35)

Day 14

Pray and ask the Lord to speak to you. Read these verses out loud then answer the questions.
"Let the peace of Christ rule in your hearts, since as members of one body you were called to peace. And be thankful. Let the message of Christ dwell among you richly as you teach and admonish one another with all wisdom through psalms, hymns, and songs from the Spirit, singing to God with gratitude in your hearts. And whatever you do, whether in word or deed, do it all in the name of the Lord Jesus, giving thanks to God the Father through him." (Col. 3:15-17)

"Let not mercy and truth forsake you; bind them around your neck, write them on the tablet of your heart, and so find favor and high esteem in the sight of God and man. Trust in the Lord with all your heart, and lean not on your own understanding; in all your ways acknowledge Him, and He shall direct your paths. It will be health to your flesh, and strength to your bones." (Prov. 3:3-6, 8)

"You will keep him in perfect peace, whose mind is stayed on You, because he trusts in You." (Isa. 26:3)

"Since we are receiving a kingdom that cannot be shaken, let us be thankful, and so worship God acceptably with reverence and awe." (Heb. 12:28) "Whoever would love life and see good days must keep their tongue from evil and their lips from deceitful speech. They must turn from evil and do good; they must seek peace and pursue it." (1 Pet. 3:10-11) "Everyone who hears these words of mine and puts them into practice is like a wise man who built his house on the rock. The rain came down, the streams rose, and the winds blew and beat against that house; yet it did not fall, because it had its foundation on the rock. But everyone who hears these words of mine and does not put them into practice is like a foolish man who built his house on sand. The rain came down, the streams rose, and the winds blew and beat against that house, and it fell with a great crash." (Matt. 7:24-27)

- How does being thankful help you to live at peace with others and stand on a strong foundation?
- Is your heart at peace right now? What is the key to keeping the peace of Christ in your heart?
- Why is God calling you to the place of peace and being thankful?
- What must you do to seek and pursue peace?
- How do you receive favor with God and man?
- What words can you speak to acknowledge God in all your ways?
- What words can you speak that will bring health to your body and strength to your bones?
- What does God want to give you through singing and thanking Him?
- How did you help and encourage someone recently with words of wisdom from God?
- What will giving thanks with your words and actions do for your health?
- When you are with someone whose words and actions are negative, how does it affect your health?
- When storms and struggles come in your life, what is the tool needed for a strong foundation, one that is unshakable?
- What Scripture verses of truth keep you from being shaken and worshipping the Lord, free from falling into complaining, arguing, or fear?

GIVE THANKS
RELEASING GOD'S POWER TO BE WHOLE

AS YOU GO
As you go through your day, focus your mind on all the MANY amazing blessings you've received through God's love and mercy, and how grateful you are for Jesus. Smile, shine God's glory, and give thanks to people for something at least 4x a day.

AFFIRMATION:
Whatever I do, whether with my words or actions, I do it all in the name of the Lord Jesus by simply giving thanks to God the Father through him and the peace of Christ rules my heart! God keeps me in perfect peace, because my mind stays on Him, trusts in Him.

LIVING FOOD VERSES DEAD FOOD

"Death and life are in the power of the tongue, and those who love it and indulge it will eat its fruit and bear the consequences of their words." "The word of God is living and powerful." (Prov. 18:21; Heb. 4:12)

Each cell of the body is like a tiny battery, and raw and living foods supply the bio-electricity which charges these batteries.

When you eat cooked (enzymeless) foods, you put a heavy burden on your body, which then has to produce the enzymes missing in the food. One of the reasons you feel lethargic or sleepy after a cooked meal is because the body is diverting its energy to replacing the enzymes that were not supplied. By comparison, a raw food meal leaves you feeling light and full of energy.

Ingesting cooked food also causes the body to produce a surge of white blood cells (leukocytosis). These cells normally defend against disease, infection, and injury to the body, but their production is a routine effect of ingesting cooked foods (as if the body considers such food a threat or danger).

Raw foods are full of oxygen, especially green leafy vegetables, which contain an abundance of chlorophyll. Chlorophyll detoxifies the bloodstream and every other part of the body better than anything else you could eat.

Sprouted seeds contain vital elements, which nourish our glands, nerves, and brain.

Raw fiber has the ability to act as a broom, which sweeps the intestinal tract and keeps it clean. Cooked fiber has lost the ability to do this for us. Enemas and colonics serve their purpose, but they are a poor substitute for what nature, by putting (raw) fiber into foods, has provided.

"Blessed are those who hunger and thirst for righteousness for they will be filled." "So whether you eat or drink or whatever you do, do it all for the glory of God." (Matt. 5:6; 1 Cor. 10:31)

Day 15

Welcome to your soup week and your last week of the challenge!
Don't forget to continue your 8 glasses of water and your smoothie as you now add soup for lunch each day. Here's an easy soup recipe, but feel free to pick any vegetable bean soup recipe.

I make it in my crockpot. 1 cup lentils, 1 cup black beans, 1 can tomato sauce, 1 small can of tomato paste, cut up celery, and lots of shaved carrots. You can put more veggies in if you like it thicker. If you like other veggies or more veggies, you could put in green, red, or yellow pepper or sweet potato. Use one box of vegetable broth, cumin and oregano. I sauté onions and garlic then put it in my crockpot. Everything else I put in and let cook. There are lots of recipes online for vegetable bean soup, so this is just a suggestion.

Pray and ask the Lord to speak to you. Read these verses out loud then answer the questions.
"Consider it pure joy, my brothers and sisters, whenever you face trials of many kinds, because you know that the testing of your faith produces perseverance. Let perseverance finish its work so that you may be mature and complete, not lacking anything." (James 1:2-4)

"We know that in all things God works for the good of those who love him, who have been called according to his purpose." (Rom. 8:28)

"Devote yourselves to prayer, being watchful and thankful." (Col. 4:2)

"Finally, my fellow believers, continue to rejoice and delight in the Lord. To write the same things again is no trouble for me, and it is a safeguard for you." (Phil. 3:1)

"The crowd joined in the attack against Paul and Silas, and the magistrates ordered them to be stripped and beaten with rods. After they had been severely flogged, they were thrown into prison, and the jailer was commanded to guard them carefully. When he received these orders, he put them in the inner cell and fastened their feet in the stocks. About midnight Paul and Silas were praying and singing hymns to God, and the other prisoners were listening to them. Suddenly there was such a violent earthquake that the foundations of the prison were shaken. At once all the prison doors flew open, and everyone's chains came loose. The jailer woke up, and when he saw the prison doors open, he drew his sword and was about to kill himself because he thought the prisoners had escaped. But Paul shouted, "Don't harm yourself! We are all here!" The jailer called for lights, rushed in and fell trembling before Paul and Silas. He then brought them out and asked, "Sirs, what must I do to be saved?" They replied, "Believe in the Lord Jesus, and you will be saved–you and your household." (Acts 16:22-31)

- **As Paul and Silas experienced being stripped, beaten with rods, severely flogged, and thrown into prison, what do you think would cause them to praise and pray in this trial?**
- **What could have been their response?**
- **How would those bad thoughts and emotions have affected them, their situation, and others around them?**
- **How can you have the same attitude of praise in your trials?**
- **When you're going through a very tough time, how can you receive God's power and breakthrough?**
- **Since your words have the power of life and death, how could death words have destroyed Paul and Silas and their ministry?**
- **How did Paul and Silas use the power of their tongues to bring freedom?**
- **How were others affected by their words?**

GIVE THANKS
RELEASING GOD'S POWER TO BE WHOLE

- Why did God add thanksgiving to devoting yourself to prayer and being watchful?
- When you know that something is dangerous, you want people to know how to stay safe from it. What thoughts and emotions that come from Satan are dangerous, and how can you be safe and free by praising and rejoicing in the Lord?
- In what area of your life do you need a breakthrough?
- When you are in bondage to something and you can't stop, what things have you tried to get free from it?
- What is God's way for you to get free from bondage?
- When you are struggling in some area, how will you lack nothing and have everything you need to come out victorious?

AS YOU GO
As you go through your day, focus your mind on all the MANY amazing blessings you've received through God's love and mercy, and how grateful you are for Jesus. Smile, shine God's glory, and give thanks to people for something at least 5x a day.

AFFIRMATION:
I consider it pure joy when I face trials, because I know that the testing of my faith to rejoice and not complain produces perseverance, matures and completes me, and I don't lack anything. I thank God always in my trials for using it for so much good in my life!

THANKFUL QUOTES
To begin this week, you could use a small chalkboard, maker board, or just use paper to write your favorite thankful quote for the day. Put it somewhere you'll be seeing it a lot so that you can focus on it many times through your day.

"Sing and make music from your heart to the Lord, always giving thanks to God the Father for everything, in the name of our Lord Jesus Christ." (Eph. 5:19-20)

"Giving thanks is one of the most loving things that you can do!"

"Feeling gratitude and not expressing it is like wrapping a present and not giving it."

"No one who achieves success does so without acknowledging the help of others."

"We would worry less if we praised more."

"Gratitude unlocks the fullness of life. It turns what we have into enough, and more. It turns denial into acceptance, chaos to order, confusion to clarity. It can turn a meal into a feast, a house into a home, a stranger into a friend." Melody Beattie

"Be thankful for what you have; you'll end up having more. If you concentrate on what you don't have, you will never, ever have enough." Oprah Winfrey

"When you rise in the morning, give thanks for the light, for your life, for your strength. Give thanks for your food and for the joy of living. If you see no reason to give thanks, the fault lies in yourself." Tecumseh

"Whatever we are waiting for–peace of mind, contentment, grace, the inner awareness of simple abundance–it will surely come to us, but only when we are ready to receive it with an open and grateful heart." Sarah Ban Breathnach

"When you are grateful–when you can see what you have–you unlock blessings to flow in your life."
Suze Orman

Day 16

Pray and ask the Lord to speak to you. Read these verses out loud then answer the questions.

"Beginning with Moses and all the Prophets, he explained to them what was said in all the Scriptures concerning himself. As they approached the village to which they were going, Jesus continued on as if he were going farther. But they urged him strongly, "Stay with us, for it is nearly evening; the day is almost over." So he went in to stay with them. When he was at the table with them, he took bread, gave thanks, broke it and began to give it to them. Then their eyes were opened and they recognized him, and he disappeared from their sight. They asked each other, "Were not our hearts burning within us while he talked with us on the road and opened the Scriptures to us?" (Luke 24:27-32)

"In the beginning was the Word, and the Word was with God, and the Word was God… Through him all things were made; without him nothing was made that has been made. In him was life, and that life was the light of all mankind. The Word (Jesus) became flesh and made his dwelling among us. We have seen his glory, the glory of the one and only Son, who came from the Father, full of grace and truth." (John 1:1-4, 14)

"For the word of God is living and powerful, and sharper than any two-edged sword, piercing even to the division of soul and spirit, and of joints and marrow, and is a discerner of the thoughts and intents of the heart." (Heb. 4:12)

"The thief comes only in order to steal and kill and destroy. I came that they may have and enjoy life, and have it in abundance [to the full, till it overflows]." (John 10:10)

"Just as you received Christ Jesus as Lord, continue to live your lives in him, rooted and built up in him, strengthened in the faith as you were taught, and overflowing with thankfulness. (Col. 2:7)

- **After Jesus was resurrected from the dead, He spoke the Scriptures to the men traveling to Emmaus. Why do you think their hearts burned when they heard Jesus speak the word of God?**
- **Words have the power of life and death. When Jesus spoke words to these men, what kind of power do you think came forth?**
- **What happens to your heart when Jesus speaks the word to you?**
- **How has the word turned on the light for you recently and revealed things that you didn't know or see?**
- **A very simple way to get free or healthy and receive God's peace and remove depression, hurt, fear, or other hard things is listening to the audio Bible. Try it and then thank the Lord for His words of life!**
- **Why did Jesus break bread and give thanks?**
- **How are you impacted when you give thanks to Jesus for His blood that was shed for you, and His body that was broken for you?**
- **What has Jesus given to you that should cause you to overflow with thanksgiving?**
- **Why should you overflow with thanksgiving for God's word daily?**
- **Since Jesus, the word, is life and light, what will His word do to your bones, joints, souls, spirit, and heart?**
- **How does the devil steal, kill, and destroy the living word from you?**
- **Why should you give thanks in everything?**

GIVE THANKS
RELEASING GOD'S POWER TO BE WHOLE

- **What will giving thanks keep you from?**
- **What will giving thanks provide for your life?**
- **How important are the words that you speak as it concerns your health and relationships?**
- **Every time that you come to the word, Jesus the bread of life, what are you expecting to receive? What is something you've received today from the word?**

AS YOU GO
As you go through your day, focus your mind on all the MANY amazing blessings you've received through God's love and mercy, and how grateful you are for Jesus. Smile, shine God's glory, and give thanks to people for something at least 5x a day.

AFFIRMATION:
I speak the word and am full of life and light. God's word makes me alive, gives me power, and gives me an abundance of life until it overflows! I overflow with thanksgiving and keep myself free and healthy!

THANKFUL QUOTES
"Sing and make music from your heart to the Lord, always giving thanks to God the Father for everything, in the name of our Lord Jesus Christ." (Eph. 5:19-20)

"The thankful receiver bears a plentiful harvest." William Blake

"Keep your eyes open to your mercies. The man who forgets to be thankful has fallen asleep in life." Robert Louis Stevenson

"None of us got to where we are alone. Whether the assistance we received was obvious or subtle, acknowledging someone's help is a big part of understanding the importance of saying thank you." Harvey Mackay

"When it comes to life, the critical thing is whether you take things for granted or take them with gratitude." Gilbert K. Chesterton

"I would maintain that thanks are the highest form of thought, and that gratitude is happiness doubled by wonder." Gilbert K. Chesterton

"Be thankful for your new identity in Christ, who you have become, and your eyes will open wider every day to the mysteries of God and the abundance of grace that's yours."

"Beginning each day with a grateful heart makes the rest of the day a thankful day."

"One of the greatest gifts you can give someone is thanking them with a sincere heart."

"Happiness comes when you stop complaining about the troubles you have and offer thanks for all the blessings of God that are yours in Christ."

"The best way to be happy is to turn the negatives into positives. You can keep the joy of the Lord as your strength by giving thanks in everything."

Pick out your favorite thankful quote for today, write it down on a paper, and keep it somewhere you can access it often. Read it many times through your day.

GIVE THANKS
RELEASING GOD'S POWER TO BE WHOLE

Day 17

Pray and ask the Lord to speak to you. Read these verses out loud then answer the questions.

"Jesus said to them all, "If anyone desires to come after Me, let him deny himself, and take up his cross daily, and follow Me. For whoever desires to save his life will lose it, but whoever loses his life for My sake will save it. For what profit is it to a man if he gains the whole world, and is himself destroyed or lost?" (Luke 9:23-25)

"I am the vine; you are the branches. If you remain in me and I in you, you will bear much fruit; apart from me you can do nothing. If you remain in me and my words remain in you, ask whatever you wish, and it will be done for you. This is to my Father's glory, that you bear much fruit, showing yourselves to be my disciples." (John 15:5, 7-8)

"Whatever you do, whether in word or deed, do it all in the name of the Lord Jesus, giving thanks to God the Father through him." (Col. 3:17)

"Let the one who boasts boast in the Lord." (2 Cor. 10:17)

"Jesus answered, "It is written: 'Man shall not live on bread alone, but on every word that comes from the mouth of God." (Matt. 4:4)

"Because you did not serve the Lord your God with joy and gladness of heart, for the abundance of everything, therefore you shall serve your enemies." (Deut. 28:47-48a)

"This is the day the Lord has made; we will rejoice and be glad in it." Psa. (118:24)

- **There's only one-way to follow Jesus and be saved (whole, healed, free) - what is it?**
- **Why will you be destroyed, lose your life, if you don't follow Jesus?**
- **If life and death are in the power of your words, how do the words you speak either cause you to keep your life and lose it, or follow Jesus and save it?**
- **What will be the results when you remain in Jesus and His word remains in you?**
- **What verse has recently held you up and made you strong through a difficult time?**
- **If giving thanks in everything is the only way to do things in Jesus' name, how can you live a life of gratitude and save your life?**
- **What did Jesus live on? Why?**
- **What does He want you to live on? Why?**
- **How do you serve the Lord?**
- **Can you serve the Lord apart from thanksgiving?**
- **What happens if you don't serve the Lord with thanksgiving?**
- **Celebrating what the Lord has done daily is the only way to give up your life. What is hindering you from giving thanks in everything?**

AS YOU GO
As you go through your day, focus your mind on all the MANY amazing blessings you've received through God's love and mercy, and how grateful you are for Jesus. Smile, shine God's glory, and give thanks to people for something at least 5x a day.

AFFIRMATION:

This is the day the Lord has made; I will serve Him with a grateful heart and rejoice for the abundance of everything I am and have in Christ! I remain in Jesus and His words remain in me His word in me, and I ask whatever I wish, and it will be done for me!

THANKFUL QUOTES

"Sing and make music from your heart to the Lord, always giving thanks to God the Father for everything, in the name of our Lord Jesus Christ." (Eph. 5:19-20)

"Gratitude delivers you from the past, brings peace for today, and gives you high expectation for tomorrow."

"Being grateful for people is showing respect and giving people honor."

"Whatever you need–peace of mind, contentment, grace, abundance of anything–it will surely come to you as you receive it with an open and grateful heart."

"The key to order, sanity, peace of mind, love, joy, and an abundance of God's goodness all comes through a grateful heart and a mouth that thanks God always in everything."

"When you are grateful for what you have, you stop complaining and start solving problems."

"Being a thankful person will always make it easy to find and keep friends, find joy, create, and be used mightily by God."

"There's no happier person than a truly thankful, content person." Joyce Meyer

"Giving thanks in everything causes the glory to go up to God and the blessings to fall down on you."

"No duty in God's eyes is more important than that of returning thanks for His indescribable gift of Jesus."

"You are really living and become radiantly alive every time you express thanks and realize all the great gifts you have to enjoy that God has freely given you."

Pick out your favorite thankful quote for today, write it down on a paper, and keep it somewhere you can access it often. Read it many times through your day.

GIVE THANKS
RELEASING GOD'S POWER TO BE WHOLE

Day 18

Pray and ask the Lord to speak to you. Read these verses out loud then answer the questions.
"Why am I discouraged? Why is my heart so sad? I will put my hope in God! I will praise him again–
my Savior and my God!" (Ps. 56:10-22)

"In God, whose word I praise, in the Lord, whose word I praise, in God I trust; I shall not be afraid.
What can man do to me?" (Psa. 42:11)

"Even when there was no reason for hope, Abraham kept hoping–believing that he would become the
father of many nations. For God had said to him, "That's how many descendants you will have!" And
Abraham's faith did not weaken, even though, at about 100 years of age, he figured his body was as
good as dead—and so was Sarah's womb. Abraham never wavered in believing God's promise. In fact,
his faith grew stronger, and in this he brought glory to God. He was fully convinced that God is able to
do whatever he promises." (Rom. 4:18-21)

"Trust in the Lord, and do good; dwell in the land, and feed on His faithfulness. Delight yourself also in
the Lord, and He shall give you the desires of your heart. Commit your way to the Lord, trust also in
Him, and He shall bring it to pass." (Psa. 37:3-5)

"He gives power to the weak and strength to the powerless. Even youths will become weak and tired,
and young men will fall in exhaustion. But those who trust (hope) in the Lord will find new strength.
They will soar high on wings like eagles. They will run and not grow weary. They will walk and not
faint." (Isa. 40:29-31)

"I pray that God, the source of hope, will fill you completely with joy and peace because you trust in
him. Then you will overflow with confident hope through the power of the Holy Spirit." (Rom. 15:13)

"In those days you were living apart from Christ.... you did not know the covenant promises God had
made. You lived in this world without God and without hope" (Eph. 2:12)

Biblical hope means to place confidence in; to trust in with confident expectation of good. It is hope
founded on God's gracious promises.

- **When you struggle with discouragement and sadness, what does God's word say is the reason?**
- **How can you be filled with hope, high expectation of good things?**
- **How are you trusting in God through His word for things in your life?**
- **What is the only way to overcome fear?**
- **Which verse from above can you put your trust in that will fill you with the most hope?**
- **How did Abraham's faith and hope grow strong and bring God's promise into His life?**
- **How does Abraham's faith and hope encourage and help you to be strengthened in your faith in a hopeless situation?**
- **What are you confident that God will bring to pass as you delight yourself in Him, trusting in His promise, and committing it to Him?**
- **How does receiving God's strength and power and putting your trust in Him relate to praying with thanksgiving?**
- **What will God fill you with right now when you trust in Him and believe His word, not what you see or feel?**

- **What things are you living apart from when you are living apart from Christ and His promises?**

AS YOU GO

As you go through your day, focus your mind on all the MANY amazing blessings you've received through God's love and mercy, and how grateful you are for Jesus. Smile, shine God's glory, and give thanks to people for something at least 5x a day.

AFFIRMATION:

I feed on God's faithfulness, delight myself in the Lord, and He gives me the desires of my heart. I commit my ways to the Lord and trust in Him, giving thanks in everything, and He shall bring it to pass.

THANKFUL QUOTES

"Sing and make music from your heart to the Lord, always giving thanks to God the Father for everything, in the name of our Lord Jesus Christ." (Eph. 5:19-20)

"The only way out of despair and tragedy is by appreciating God, others, and life. The more you express thanksgiving, the happier and healthier you become."

"When you don't have gratitude in your heart, there's a hole in your heart and you feel empty, lost, without purpose; but when you express thanks, you are filled with good things and spring to life."

Thanking God for new mercies every day is the only way to keep yourself from falling and failing, and allowing his mercy to make you alive."

"Anyone can complain or criticize. You become a hero by giving thanks in everything and make life special for everyone."

"Being thankful for the little things each day make you realize that the little things are actually the big things."

"Giving thanks to God is recognizing His goodness in your life, keeping you from the evil one, and seeing God as more precious than silver and more costly than gold."

"You'll see everyone and everything in life differently every time you express thanks for something. When you're thanking God for every little meal, drink of water, health, eyes to see, and so on, your heart begins to overflow with gratitude and appreciation."

"The gift of 'thank you' to people is one of the most precious gems in life."

Pick out your favorite thankful quote for today, write it down on a paper, and keep it somewhere you can access it often. Read it many times through your day.

Day 19

Pray and ask the Lord to speak to you. Read these verses out loud then answer the questions.
"Praise the Lord, you his servants; praise the name of the Lord. Let the name of the Lord be praised, both now and forevermore. From the rising of the sun to the place where it sets, the name of the Lord is to be praised." (Psa. 113:1-3)

"A man will be satisfied with good from the fruit of his words." (Prov. 12:14)

"He has sent me to heal the brokenhearted, to proclaim freedom for the captives and release from darkness for the prisoners... to bestow on them a crown of beauty instead of ashes, the oil of joy instead of mourning, and a garment of praise instead of a spirit of despair." (Isa. 61:1-3)

"God resists the proud, but gives grace to the humble. Therefore submit to God. Resist the devil and he will flee from you. Draw near to God and He will draw near to you." (James 4:6-8)

"Pride goes before destruction, and a haughty spirit before a fall." (Prov. 16:18)

"Now yield and submit yourself to Him [agree with God and be conformed to His will] and be at peace; in this way [you will prosper and great] good will come to you." (Job 22:21)

- **What are the good things you will be satisfied with by using your mouth to praise the Lord?**
- **What sin, bad habits, and destructive things will you avoid and break free from by using your mouth to thank and praise the Lord?**
- **God sent Jesus to heal your broken heart, give you freedom, and release you from darkness. What did He set you free from and what did He replace it with?**
- **By opening your mouth and praising the Lord, what things would you like to begin overcoming with God's grace?**
- **What does wearing praise crown you with?**
- **How does the world view submission?**
- **How can submitting to God's will of giving thanks in everything lavish you with blessings in your health and relationships?**
- **What does God promise to give you when you submit to Him and come near to Him?**
- **God's grace freely supplies all your needs, so when you submit and give thanks to God, what good emotions and thoughts will you experience?**
- **When you have bad emotions and are struggling, what is the easy solution to your problem?**
- **How is thanksgiving and praise a way of escape from pride?**
- **How does not being humble and thankful harm your relationships? How does it help them?**

AS YOU GO
As you go through your day, focus your mind on all the MANY amazing blessings you've received through God's love and mercy and how grateful you are for Jesus. Smile, shine God's glory and give thanks to people for something at least 5x a day.

AFFIRMATION:
I submit to God in everything and give Him thanks and receive an abundance of grace to meet my needs. I fill my mouth with good by giving thanks and am satisfied with lots of good things.

THANKFUL QUOTES
"Sing and make music from your heart to the Lord, always giving thanks to God the Father for everything, in the name of our Lord Jesus Christ." (Eph. 5:19-20)

"Give thanks every day for God's love being poured into your heart and you will discover a new life of love that will radically change your life."

"You can choose every day to see the problem or the multitude of abundant blessings you've received in Christ."

"Attitude is everything, and having a thankful attitude puts you at the highest level of living."

"Happiness isn't about getting more. It's about loving what you have and being grateful for it."

"A grateful heart is a magnet for miracles. Expressing thanks is the quickest way to see change in any area of your life."

"Replacing expectation with gratitude brings great results."

"Giving thanks in everything is celebrating the little things in life; it takes you higher and to bigger things in life."

"I found out after years of stumbling daily over my own feet that I had the key to a life more abundant through thanksgiving."

"Kindness releases God's power and giving thanks is the way to kindness."

"A great gift of gratitude is that the more grateful you are, the more present you become and living in the moment is making everything special, fun, and enjoyable."

Pick out your favorite thankful quote for today, write it down on a paper, and keep it somewhere you can access it often. Read it many times through your day.

GIVE THANKS
RELEASING GOD'S POWER TO BE WHOLE

Day 20

Pray and ask the Lord to speak to you. Read these verses out loud then answer the questions.
"No temptation has overtaken you except what is common to mankind. And God is faithful; he will not let you be tempted beyond what you can bear. But when you are tempted, he will also provide a way out so that you can endure it." (1 Cor. 10:13)

"Follow God's example, therefore, as dearly loved children and walk in the way of love, just as Christ loved us and gave himself up for us as a fragrant offering and sacrifice to God. But among you there must not be even a hint of sexual immorality, or of any kind of impurity, or of greed, because these are improper for God's holy people. Nor should there be obscenity, foolish talk or coarse joking, which are out of place, but rather thanksgiving." (Eph. 5:1-4)

"Do not be overcome by evil, but overcome evil with good." (Rom. 12:21)

"You are my God, and I will give you thanks; you are my God, and I will exalt you. Give thanks to the LORD, for he is good; his love endures forever." (Psa. 118:28-29)

"Do not let any unwholesome talk come out of your mouths, but what is good for necessary edification, that it may impart grace to the hearers. And do not grieve the Holy Spirit of God ... Let all bitterness, wrath, anger, clamor, and evil speaking be put away from you, with all malice. And be kind to one another, tenderhearted, forgiving one another, even as God in Christ forgave you." (Eph. 4:29-32)

- **You've seen lepers get healed and one made whole, Jonah find salvation from death in a fish, Jehoshaphat find freedom from a vast army, Paul find breakthrough in prison, and Jesus bringing life to a dead person! What was their way of escape, success, and victory?**
- **What is your secret to be successful in your relationships, health, job, and ministry?**
- **What things tempt you to complain rather than give thanks to God?**
- **How can you overcome the temptation of arguing, negative speaking, and complaining?**
- **How does it help you knowing all the benefits, protection, provision, peace, and God's presence of life that you receive through giving thanks?**
- **How do you walk in love and avoid the evil attitudes, thoughts, and desires?**
- **What are the good things that you can do to overcome any kind of evil?**
- **Hebrews 12:15 says that bitterness defiles you. What's God's way for you to overcome and escape bitterness quickly?**
- **Why does God want you to forgive?**
- **How does God want you to forgive others?**
- **What good words of truth has God given you to think, believe, and speak to overcome and escape from evil such as fear, anger, doubt, hurt, lust, etc?**
- **What unwholesome words are you able to overcome through a daily habit of thanksgiving and praise?**

AS YOU GO
As you go through your day, focus your mind on all the MANY amazing blessings you've received through God's love and mercy, and how grateful you are for Jesus. Smile, shine God's glory, and give thanks to people for something at least 5x a day.

AFFIRMATION:

I overcome evil with good and keep all unwholesome talk from coming out my mouth by giving thanks in everything. I speak wholesome words of kindness and tenderheartedness, and forgive others, even as God in Christ forgave me by keeping a thankful attitude.

THANKFUL QUOTES

"Sing and make music from your heart to the Lord, always giving thanks to God the Father for everything, in the name of our Lord Jesus Christ." (Eph. 5:19-20)

"Gratitude is the open door to abundance."

"Showing gratitude is one of the simplest yet most powerful things humans can do for each other." - Randy Pausch

"Giving thanks to people opens their eyes to the gifts God has given them and helps them grow stronger in their real self."

"It isn't what you have in your pocket that makes you thankful, but what you have in your heart, Jesus, the Bread of life!"

"When you magnify Jesus instead of magnifying disappointments, you will experience the fullness of joy."

Life is not about getting, but being a giver and giving thanks in everything, which makes your life amazing, wonderful, and a blessing everyday."

"You can give without loving, but you cannot love without giving." -Amy Carmichael

"Thanksgiving is one of the greatest forms of showing love."

"It's by giving that you receive good things, and when you give thanks to God, you lack no good thing and have everything you need for life."

"Every time we remember to say "thank you", we experience nothing less than heaven on earth." -Sarah Ban Breathnach

Pick out your favorite thankful quote for today, write it down on a paper, and keep it somewhere you can access it often. Read it many times through your day.

GIVE THANKS
RELEASING GOD'S POWER TO BE WHOLE

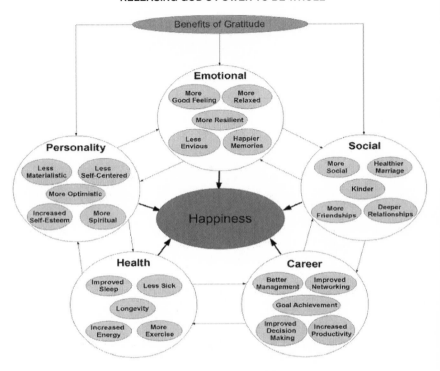

Day 21

Pray and ask the Lord to speak to you. Read these verses out loud then answer the questions.

"Today I have given you the choice between life and death, between blessings and curses. Oh, that you would choose life, so that you and your descendants might live! You can make this choice by loving the Lord your God, obeying him, and committing yourself firmly to him. This is the key to your life." (Deut. 30:19-20)

"Let the one who boasts boast in the Lord." (1 Cor. 1:31)

"Giving thanks is a sacrifice that truly honors me. If you keep to my path, I will reveal to you the salvation of God." (Psa. 50:23)

"The thief does not come except to steal, and to kill, and to destroy. I have come that they may have life, and that they may have it more abundantly." (John 10:10)

"Therefore, I urge you, brothers and sisters, in view of God's mercy, to offer your bodies as a living sacrifice, holy and pleasing to God–this is your true and proper worship. Do not conform to the pattern of this world, but be transformed by the renewing of your mind…" (Rom. 12:1-2)

"My thoughts are nothing like your thoughts," says the Lord. And my ways are far beyond anything you could imagine. For just as the heavens are higher than the earth, so my ways are higher than your ways and my thoughts higher than your thoughts." (Isa. 55:8-9)

"If anyone is in Christ, he is a new creation; old things have passed away; behold, all things have become new." (2 Cor. 5:17)

"For the law of the Spirit of life in Christ Jesus has made me free from the law of sin and death. For those who live according to the flesh set their minds on the things of the flesh, but those who live according to the Spirit, have their minds set on the things of the Spirit. For to be carnally minded is death, but to be spiritually minded is life and peace." (Rom. 8:2, 5-6)

"It is good to give thanks to the Lord, to sing praises to the Most High. It is good to proclaim your unfailing love in the morning, your faithfulness in the evening." (Psa. 92:1-2)

- **What two choices does God's word say that you have?**
- **How do you choose life daily?**
- **Which choice do you think is related to giving thanks in everything, and which one to complaining and arguing?**
- **Every day you get to choose whether to sacrifice your thoughts and ways of complaining for His thoughts and ways of thanksgiving. Why is giving thanks considered a sacrifice?**
- **How do you become a living sacrifice?**
- **Have you ever experienced a miracle, strength, healing, or other blessings through sacrificing your mouth to give thanks when it was the last thing you felt like doing?**
- **What would cause you to not want to give thanks in everything and do God's will and have life, which is blessings of every kind, and life more abundantly?**
- **When others choose to complain and argue, how can you help them to choose life?**
- **How different are God's thoughts and ways than yours?**
- **How different is the way that you handle an angry, complaining person than the way God handles them?**

- **What kind of thoughts do you think will take you to high living, an abundant life, and which ones to low living, death?**
- **How many of your thoughts and words become new in Christ?**
- **How serious should you consider your thought life?**
- **How do you choose to set your mind on something?**
- **Why do you think giving thanks and praise to God is a good thing?**
- **Do you see how you were created for God and how words connect you to Him and release the power of life through your mouth? Words really do have the power of life and death. What a gift you've been given through your words of thanksgiving and praise to God!**

AS YOU GO

As you go through your day, focus your mind on all the MANY amazing blessings you've received through God's love and mercy, and how grateful you are for Jesus. Smile, shine God's glory, and give thanks to people for something at least 5x a day.

AFFIRMATION:

I give thanks and sacrifice to the Lord and truly honor Him, keep to His path, and He will reveal to me His salvation. It is good for me to give thanks to the Lord, to sing praises to the Most High. It is good for me to proclaim His unfailing love in the morning and His faithfulness in the evening!

THANKFUL QUOTES

"Sing and make music from your heart to the Lord, always giving thanks to God the Father for everything, in the name of our Lord Jesus Christ." (Eph. 5:19-20)

"The thankful receiver bears a plentiful harvest." – William Blake

"Gratitude is not only the greatest of virtues, but the parent of all the others." – Marcus Tullius Cicero

"Only a fool refuses to give thanks and ends up in a pit of darkness. Thanksgiving is the key to receiving all of God's blessings. Thanksgiving puts you in the light and light always overcomes darkness."

"Gratitude makes every moment purposeful and powerful. Giving thanks to God in everything is a choice that makes the most amazing difference in every area of your life."

"Being thankful can make us happy and at the same time, we can learn to appreciate the things that we have."

"The real gift of gratitude is that the more grateful you are, the more present you become." -Robert Holden

"When we focus on our gratitude, the tide of disappointment goes out and the tide of love rushes in." - Kristin Armstrong

"Gratitude can transform common days into thanksgiving, turn routine jobs into joy and change ordinary opportunities into blessings." -William Arthur Ward

"God gave you a gift of 84,600 seconds today. Have you used one of them to say thank you?" -William Arthur Ward

"There is always supernatural provision available for us, when we connect to God through thanksgiving."

"God is able to do exceedingly abundantly above all that we ask or think when we put ourselves under His love and care and give thanks in everything."

"Thanksgiving empowers you with faith and faith moves and pleases God."

"A grateful heart and a mouth full of thanksgiving gives you a healthy, free heart and life, one that is overflowing with abundance of good things, and one that enjoys God and people."

"There is a calmness to a life lived in gratitude, a quiet joy." – Ralph Blum

"No duty is more urgent than that of returning thanks." –James Allen

"If it is received with gratitude; it is sanctified [set apart, dedicated to God] by means of the word of God and prayer." (1 Tim. 4:4-5)

"God says to not be anxious about anything, but in everything pray with thanksgiving. But we think praying to God is first, and then wait to see results before giving thanks to Him. God is good and His love endures forever, and He loves to give good things to His children!"

Thanksgiving OVERCOMES greed, selfishness, pride, anger, bitterness, addictions, lust, fear, depression, despair, loneliness, jealousy, envy, confusion – all evil and brings life, which is health and freedom. Giving thanks is the one thing that can overcome many things! Thanksgiving covers a multitude of sin! Give thanks and live free and healthy!

Pick out your favorite thankful quote for today, write it down on a paper, and keep it somewhere you can access it often. Read it many times through your day.

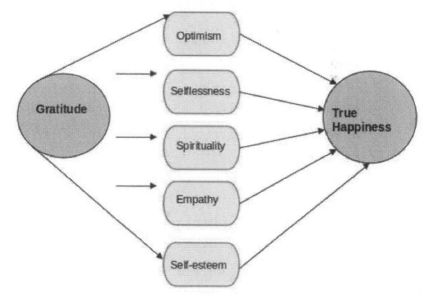

GIVE THANKS
RELEASING GOD'S POWER TO BE WHOLE

May you never forget that you have the power of God available in every area your life through giving thanks! Here are words to say to yourself daily and keep you remembering and enjoying all the blessings of God.

"My mouth is controlling my body and my life."
"I live God's way of giving thanks to Him in everything which is the way of all that's good, pleasing, and perfect!"
"Giving thanks will always bless and prosper me, and always heal and free me!"
"I will always find rest, peace, and joy, and always bring extremely wonderful things to my health and relationships by giving thanks always!"
"I give thanks to God in everything and avoid a multitude of sin and receive an abundance of life!"

Giving thanks will release God's power in your life, and you will be whole!

Made in the USA
Columbia, SC
02 January 2020

86170306R00033